EMA BALOS

What to Expect in Labor

A Comprehensive Guide to Coping Techniques for Each Stage of Labor

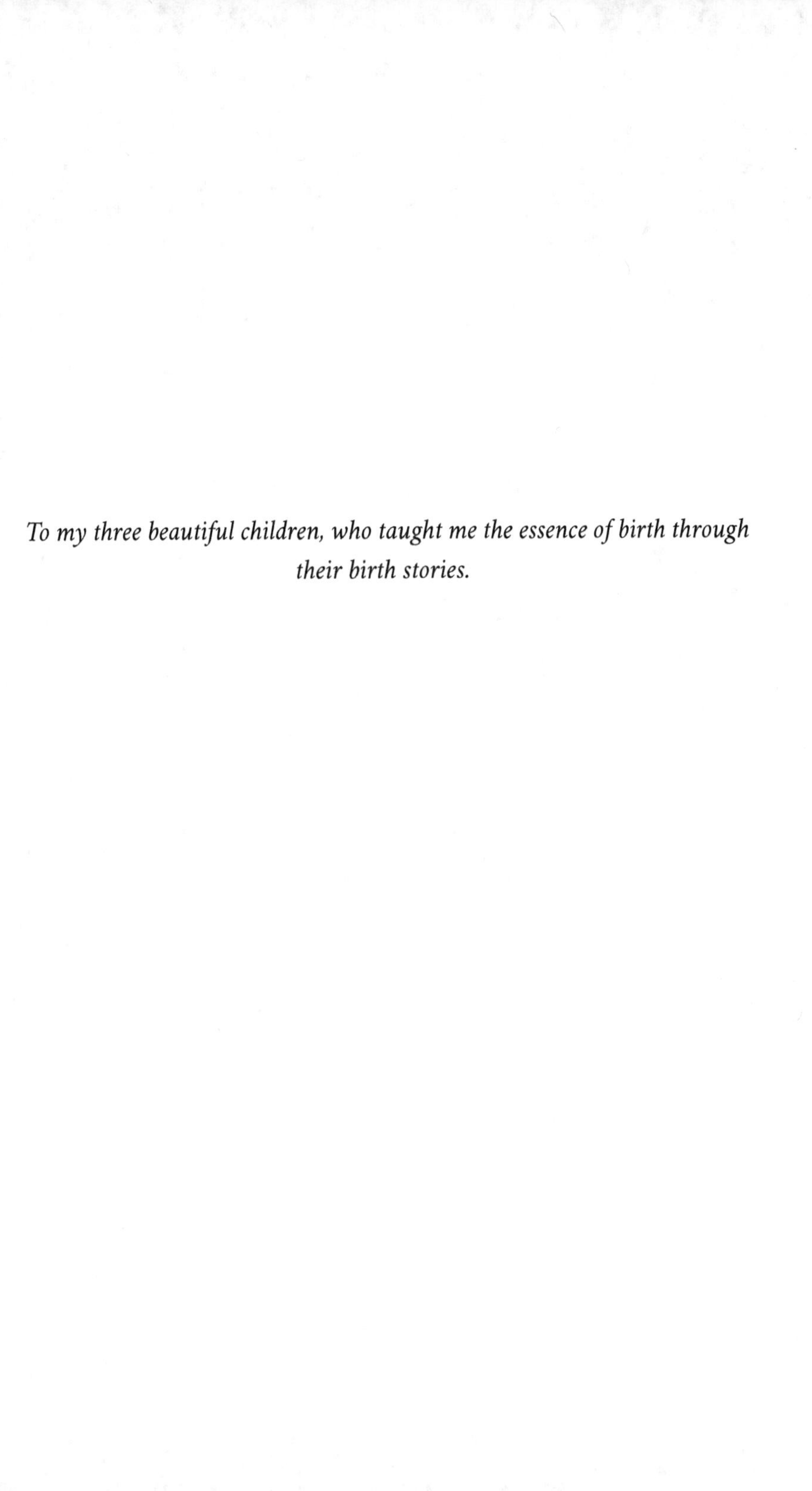

To my three beautiful children, who taught me the essence of birth through their birth stories.

"You gain strength, courage, and confidence by every experience in which you
really stop and look fear in the face"

-ELEANOR ROOSEVELT

Contents

1

Your Empowered Birth Awaits

Bringing a new life into the world is an extraordinary journey, one filled with both awe-inspiring moments and challenges that test the limits of body, mind, and heart. Labor, the pivotal passage from pregnancy to parenthood, is an experience that no two people will navigate quite the same way. It's a unique blend of strength, vulnerability, and resilience, and it's during this transformative process that the depth of your own capabilities becomes evident.

In "What to Expect in Labor: A Comprehensive Guide to Coping Techniques for Each Stage of Labor," we embark on a holistic exploration of the stages of labor, offering you a road map to navigate the challenges that lie ahead with confidence and grace. Throughout this book, I, your virtual birth doula, share a profound understanding of the physical, emotional, and mental aspects of labor, and the invaluable role that your support team will play in helping you achieve a positive birth experience.

This book is designed to give you very practical guidance offering very specific coping techniques for each stage of labor. It's designed to empower your birth, giving you the confidence and courage to step into birth feeling educated and equipped.

The Stages of Labor

Labor unfolds in distinct stages: early labor, active labor, and the pushing stage, each presenting its own unique demands. We delve into the intricacies of these phases, guiding you through the physical sensations, the emotional fluctuations, and the mental fortitude needed to progress through labor. With the right coping techniques, you'll discover how to harness your inner strength and adapt to the evolving needs of each stage.

Coping with Your Whole Self: Body, Mind, and Heart

Labor is an all-encompassing experience, involving not just your body, but your mind and heart as well. "What to Expect in Labor" recognizes this holistic approach and provides a comprehensive toolkit for coping with your whole self. We will explore the physical techniques that help manage pain and discomfort, the mental strategies that strengthen your resolve, and the emotional support that ensures your heart remains resilient throughout.

Physical Coping Techniques

The body is a powerful instrument, capable of enduring the demands of labor when equipped with the right coping techniques. This book will guide you through movement, relaxation, massage, and position changes that can alleviate discomfort and facilitate labor progression. You'll discover how to work with your body, not against it, to achieve a smoother and more comfortable birth.

Emotional Coping Techniques

We explore the array of emotions that labor can evoke, from anticipation and excitement to moments of doubt and fear. You'll learn to navigate these feelings through mindfulness, breathing exercises, visualization, and positive affirmations. "What to Expect in Labor" offers a wealth of emotional coping strategies to help you maintain a sense of calm, confidence, and empowerment.

Mental Coping Techniques

Your mental resilience is a cornerstone of successful labor. We explore techniques for maintaining focus, reducing anxiety, and staying present throughout the process. With mindfulness and guided imagery, you'll develop the mental strength required to navigate the peaks and valleys of labor.

The Role of Support People: Partner and Birth Doula

In addition to your own inner strength, the presence of your partner and a skilled birth doula can make a profound difference. We outline the pivotal role they play in supporting you emotionally, providing physical comfort, and advocating for your birth preferences. With their assistance, you'll forge an unbreakable bond that fosters a sense of trust, unity, and empowerment.

"What to Expect in Labor" is not just a guide; it's a companion on your journey to parenthood. It's a testament to the incredible capacity within you and a testament to the power of your support system. Together, we'll unlock the potential for a birth experience that is not only safe and positive but deeply empowering.

2

Early Labor: The Power of Rest

Early labor – the initial stage of your remarkable journey of labor– is a time of gentle anticipation. It's a moment to savor and a phase to embrace with a sense of calm and assurance. In this chapter, we will explore the art of managing early labor, a phase that sets the stage for the beautiful and transformative moments that lie ahead. As a seasoned guide in the field of childbirth, my aim is to provide you with both professional insight and a touch of personal understanding, helping you approach early labor with the poise it deserves.

The Essence of Early Labor

Balance and Patience

Early labor is like the opening act of a play, setting the tone for the main performance. It is a time when contractions are typically mild and infrequent, allowing you the opportunity to maintain a semblance of normalcy in your life. At this stage, the key is to strike a balance between staying active and seeking restorative moments. Engaging in activities that act as distractions, such as a leisurely walk, preparing a simple meal, or enjoying a movie, can help take your mind off the impending labor and infuse your day with a sense of calm.

Conversely, cherish those restful interludes. A warm bath or shower can work wonders in soothing your body and calming your mind. A gentle massage, cuddling or kissing can help awaken the hormones that are delicate in this stage and need a sense of safety to build. Ideally you can sleep, even if it's in small intervals or little cat naps. Your environment plays a vital role during this phase. Set up a serene space with soft music, dim lighting, candles, and aromatherapy creating an ambiance that resonates with tranquility and peace. Your environment will help you feel safe and secure, which is vital in encouraging your body to move into the more active stage of labor.

Energy Conservation

One of the fundamental principles of early labor is the judicious preservation of energy. This stage is not the time to over-focus on labor itself but to mindfully channel your efforts into conserving your physical and emotional vitality. By alternating between distracting activities and rest, you ensure a dynamic equilibrium that sets you up beautiful for the rest of labor.

It's important to note that, in most cases, there is no immediate need to rush to the hospital or birth center during early labor, especially for a first time mom. Staying in the comfort of your home during early labor is often ideal. Home is where you feel most at ease, where your surroundings are familiar, and where your sense of security is paramount.

Embracing Oxytocin and Pleasure

Early labor is an opportune time to harness the magic of oxytocin, often referred to as the "love hormone" or "bonding hormone." This hormone plays a pivotal role in childbirth, and you can encourage its release by engaging in pleasurable activities. Kissing, cuddling with your partner, and gentle stimulation of your nipples and clitoris can promote the production of oxytocin. These activities enhance your emotional sense of well-being and provoke the hormones that help expedite the transition from early to active labor.

Embrace this phase with a sense of curiosity, adventure, and trust in your body's innate wisdom. Early labor is your invitation to savor every moment as you progress toward the pinnacle of birth. Heading to the hospital or birth center in early labor can often interrupt the gentle building of the hormones needed for contractions to intensify. It's common for labor to stall or even stop if you leave the safety and security of your comfortable home.

Early Labor: Physically

During early labor, your body undergoes subtle but significant changes in preparation for the birth of your baby. Here are some of the physical signs and sensations you might experience:

Cervical Changes: Your cervix is ripening, effacing (thinning out), and gradually moving forward, signaling the beginning of the birthing process.

Cramps and Backache: You might feel period-like cramps, an aching back, or even experience mild contractions. These sensations can be uncomfortable and may leave you feeling restless as your body readies itself.

Mucus Plug: It's not uncommon to lose your mucus plug during this phase. This jelly-like substance serves as a protective barrier for your baby, and its loss is a clear sign that labor is pending.

Restless Nights: Sleeping can become a challenge during early labor, as contractions may keep you up at night. It's important to rest when you can, as you'll need your strength as contractions begin to pick up in intensity.

Soft Stool: Some women experience loose stools during early labor, which is a natural response as your body clears the way and makes more room for baby to descend.

Contractions: You may notice mild contractions that gradually become longer, stronger, and closer together. These contractions tend to feel manageable and grow in length and intensity at a slow and steady pace. Keep in mind that it's very normal for contraction patterns to be irregular or inconsistent during this stage.

Early Labor: Emotionally

You can anticipate a range of emotions in the early stage of labor. Here are some of the emotional states you might find yourself in:

Excitement and Anticipation: You may feel elated, talkative, and even find yourself smiling in sheer anticipation, the much awaited moment of labor is here.

Restlessness and Anxiety: Mixed with excitement, restlessness and anxiety can creep in. The wonder of "Is this really it?" might be paired with nervousness about the unknown.

Energetic Yet Fearful: Paradoxically, you may feel a surge of energy while also battling fear and apprehension about what lies ahead.

The range of these emotions are all part of the emotional tapestry of early labor. It's okay to feel a mix of emotions and to give them room to come and go.

Early Labor: Your Support Team

Your partner, along with your birth doula and anyone else you have on your support team, will join you in your excitement and anticipation during early labor. Here are important and helpful ways your support team can assist you in early labor:

Hydration and Nutrition: Remind you to stay hydrated and eat often – even if it is small yet hardy snacks. Nourishing your body is vital for the energy you'll require.

Timing Contractions: Help time your contractions to gauge their frequency and intensity. I recommend timing them for 30-60 minutes and then pausing to allow you to distract yourself or rest. Staying present to the moment rather than focused on the contractions and timing them is invaluable in conserving energy. Continuous tracking of contractions is not necessary and can add unnecessary fatigue or interfere with the natural flow of labor.

Creating a Soothing Environment: Establish a calm, soothing atmosphere. Music, dim lighting, and a comforting ambiance can enhance your sense of safety and security. When you feel safe and secure you are able to let go and trust the process which will encourage labor to progress more swiftly.

Emotional Support: Listening attentively as you navigate through contractions and the emotional ebbs and flows of early labor. Offer reassurance and care to help you stay calm and excited through early labor.

Guidance on Positions: Recommendations for positions that can encourage labor progression and optimize your baby's positioning. Changing positions often will help usher labor into a more active pattern.

Continual Connection: Your partner or doula/support team can offer suggestions for distractions and emotional support. Your doula may stop by your home to help you with positions, movement and mindfulness if you feel like you need that support in early labor or if early labor is very long.

Timing for Hospital Arrival: Your support (especially a doula) can help you gauge when it's time to head to the hospital, ensuring you arrive at the right moment for a smooth transition into your new setting.

Early labor is a unique blend of physical, emotional, and mental gearing up for labor. It's a time when emotions are fragile and delicate so your environment and sense of safety and security are so important. Your body is preparing for labor to intensify, your emotions and hormones are revving up, and your support team is here to guide and empower you through this incredible and exhilarating early stage.

Having a birth doula to walk alongside you, providing professional expertise and guidance as well as empathy and care can really help shape your birth experience. A birth doula can help you feel confident and courageous, encourage you to trust your body and the process, help you navigate when it's time to go to your birth place, and be a steady source of comfort, reassurance, and empowerment.

Early Labor: Coping Techniques

Let's explore very practical techniques to help you cope through the early stage of labor. The top focus of this stage reflected in these techniques is three fold: to help you stay distracted, to help you rest to conserve energy, and to activate the hormones needed for labor.

Distractions

Watch a Movie: Lose yourself in a captivating film or one of your favorite shows to help temporarily divert your focus from the early stages of labor.

Go for a Walk(s): Take a leisurely stroll or hefty paced walk in the fresh air - go at a pace that feels comfortable to you. The rhythm of your steps can be soothing. As you are active it encourages contractions to become more active.

Make a Meal/Eat: Preparing a simple meal or enjoying a nourishing snack can provide both a physical distraction and the sustenance your body needs.

Hydrate (water, tea, electrolyte water, coconut water, laborades etc...): Stay hydrated, sipping on water, herbal tea, or hydrating beverages.

Miles Circuit* (3-Step Sequence Optimizing Baby's Position):
   #1. Open Knees, Forward Lean (30 minutes): Get on your hands and knees, allowing your knees to open wide. Lower your arms, resting on a pillow or the floor, while keeping your bottom elevated.

#2. Exaggerated Side Lying (30 minutes): Lying on your side, arch your top leg as high as you can while keeping your bottom arm and leg straight. Try to turn onto your belly as much as you can.

#3. Upright Asymmetric Position (30 minutes): Experiment with any upright asymmetric position that suits you, like lunges, stair climbing (two steps at a time), or walking with one foot on a curb. Maintain a wide and open pelvis in your chosen position.

*You can find a pdf with more detailed description of the Miles Circuit, along with visuals here: https://www.milescircuit.com/uploads/4/8/1 /4/4814341/miles_circuit.pdf

Rest

Sleep/Rest in Bed: If possible, get some sleep or rest in bed. Your body needs to conserve its strength for the more active part of labor ahead.

Listen to Music/Podcast: Choose to listen to soothing music or engage your mind with an inspiring podcast to create a calming environment.

Guided Meditation/Relaxation: Center yourself with guided meditation or relaxation exercises. Listening to guided meditations prenatally will be helpful, so when you play them in early labor it will naturally and easily trigger your mind and body to relax. If you've choose to prepare with hypnobirthing tracks, this is a great time to start listening.

Shower/Bath: Enjoy a warm shower or bath to relax your muscles and ease any discomfort. If your bag of waters has ruptured, some providers recommend waiting to use the bath until contraction patterns become more frequent.

Sit on a Birth/Yoga Ball: Find comfort by sitting on a birth or yoga ball; for added comfort let your head rest on the bed or the top part of your couch. The gentle rocking motion can be soothing and offer dynamic movement in your pelvis. Try circles, figure 8's, U-shaped or gentle bouncing to help with both comfort and to encourage progress.

Quiet Environment (i.e. Music, Diffuse Essential Oils, Dim Lights): Dim the lights, play calming music, and diffuse essential oils to create a tranquil atmosphere that will give you a sense of safety and security and encourage rest.

Solitude: Sometimes, a moment of solitude can provide solace. Reflect, meditate, or simply be with your thoughts. Solitude can also help you not feel like you are being observed, which can help you relax into your labor.

Create Physical Comfort/Relaxation (Pillows, Lying Down Runner's Pose): Arrange pillows to support your body, and consider lying in a relaxed runner's pose for physical comfort and relaxation.

Activate

These methods help activate the hormones (Oxycontin, endorphins, prolactin) essential for labor:

Spooning: Cuddle up in a spooning position with your partner, fostering a sense of intimacy and closeness.

Hugging: Share a long comforting hug with your partner. Physical touch can be incredibly reassuring during this time.

Kissing: The power of a gentle kiss can stimulate the release of oxytocin, enhancing your sense of security.

Gentle Touch: Light, tender touches from your partner or support person can soothe and reassure you.

Clitoral Stimulation: Gentle clitoral stimulation may help activate oxytocin, bringing forth those powerful labor hormones and creating a more rhythmic contraction pattern.

Nipple Stimulation: Nipple stimulation can contribute to the release of oxytocin and support the progress of labor.

Read/Repeat Positive Affirmations: Surround yourself with positive affirmations. Reading and repeating them can infuse your mind with confidence and optimism.

Each of these coping techniques can serve as valuable tools in your labor, helping you cope and stay present in the moment. During your pregnancy spend some time exploring and utilizing these techniques, that way when labor starts you can be ready to use them. It will feel natural and comforting to reach for them to help you relax, stay present, and connect with your body, your baby, and your birth - if you use the techniques throughout pregnancy.

3

Active Labor: The Power of Rhythms

Active labor is a profound passage in the birthing journey, where your body surges with strength and determination to bring your baby into the world. This chapter will serve as a guide, helping you navigate through this pivotal stage of labor, offering both professional insights and a heartfelt understanding of the emotional and physical challenges you may encounter.

In active labor, the art of rhythm takes center stage. It is the compass that will guide you through the ebbs and flows of contractions, offering you a sense of control and grounding amidst the intensity. Rhythms are your trusted companions, helping you move with grace and ease through this dynamic stage. It's within the rhythms that you'll find the power to manage the contractions and draw strength from within.

Rhythms in Active Labor

Creating Your Rhythm

Imagine your rhythm as a harmonious blend of coping techniques, carefully chosen to suit your unique needs. During active labor, select 2-4 of these techniques and bundle them together into a personalized rhythm. These rhythms will be your sanctuary through each contraction. They'll anchor you, providing a steady foundation that will enable you to navigate each contraction with poise and resilience.

As a contraction begins, reach for your rhythm. Feel it envelop you as the contraction rises and reaches its peak. Let it guide you through the waves of intensity, allowing you to focus your energy and attention where it's most needed.

In Between Contractions

The moments between contractions offer you a precious respite. Use this time wisely to rest your body and mind. As you wait for the next surge of energy, engage in the following practices:

Rest: Allow your body to rest. Sink into the comfort that comes with the break, conserving your energy for the contractions that lie ahead. All the intensity and pain of contractions subside in between contractions, take full advantage and enjoy the break.

Complete Relaxation: From the crown of your head to the tips of your toes, consciously relax each part of your body. Let tension melt away, leaving you feeling light and free and ready to take on just the next contraction.

Take Deep Cleansing Breaths: Inhale deeply, drawing in rejuvenating breaths, and exhale with purpose, releasing any lingering tension. These cleansing breaths will refresh your spirit and prepare you for the next wave.

Changing Your Rhythm

Change is the heartbeat of progress in active labor. To optimize your experience, reduce pain and expedite the birthing process, it's crucial to change your rhythm every 5-10 contractions. This deliberate shifting of your coping techniques serves multiple vital purposes:

Shorten Labor: Changing your rhythm can encourage labor to progress steadily, bringing you to the moment when you'll meet your baby sooner.

Optimal Baby Position: Different rhythms can help encourage your baby to assume the optimal position for birth, ensuring a smoother descent through the pelvis.

Avoid Labor Stalling: By introducing variety, you can help prevent labor from stalling or slowing down, maintaining a steady pace toward your baby's arrival.

Mind and Emotion Steadiness: Changing rhythms keeps your mind and emotions in the present moment, helping you stay connected to your body and your baby. Rhythms help maintain a sense of control and empowerment.

Momentum and Endurance: A change in rhythm can help sustain momentum and endurance, ensuring you remain resilient even in the most intense moments of labor.

Let's explore the best combination of coping techniques that resonate with your unique personality and preferences. Rhythms and the art of changing them frequently will anchor you through the intensity of active labor, allowing you to move forward with strength and determination. Using rhythms in labor will help you uncover the power within you, and will help guide you through active labor.

Active Labor: Physically

In the throes of active labor, your body undergoes a remarkable transformation. Here's a detailed exploration of the physical sensations and experiences that may unfold:

Cervix is dilating from 5-10 cm: The contractions of active labor continue dilating your cervix until you are completely dilated.

Bloody show: A telling sign that contractions are making good and useful change to your cervix is having discharge, often bloody and thick or mucusy.

Nausea and Vomiting: Some women may experience nausea or even vomit during active labor. These are common responses as your body is feeling the intensity of contractions.

Emotional Variability: The physical intensity is often mirrored by emotional fluctuations. You might find yourself feeling weepy, shaky, or on edge. These emotional variations are entirely normal as you navigate the intensity of active labor. This sometimes comes with shaking, you're typically not cold but your body is shaking.

Fluctuating Body Temperature: You may alternate between feeling hot and cold. It's a response to the powerful surge of energy your body is generating.

Loss of Appetite: It's common to lose your appetite or have a reduced desire to eat or drink. However, taking small bites and sips is a good idea to maintain your energy levels.

Contractions Taking Center Stage: Contractions become the focal point of your attention. You'll pause and focus, moving inward as each contraction ebbs and flows.

Increased Need for Movement: The urge to move intensifies as your body adapts to the demands of labor. Shifting positions and staying mobile can provide relief and facilitate progress.

Vocalization: Many women find that vocalizing or making sounds feels natural and helpful. It can be a valuable coping mechanism during the intensity of contractions.

Baby's Descent: As your baby descends, contractions continue to grow closer, longer, and stronger. This progression is a significant sign that things are moving forward well.

Baby's Position: If your baby is in a less favorable position, labor may appear to slow down or stall as your baby attempts to reposition. If baby is positioned head down but facing mom's abdominal, baby is Occiput

Posterior (OP) — this can create 'back labor' and can create stronger back pain through labor (about 30% of mom's experience this kind of labor). Frequent changes in your own position can help encourage the baby to find a more optimal alignment.

Ruptured Membranes/Water Breaking: At this stage, your water may break if it has not already. This can happen suddenly with a pop and a gush or occur as a gradual leak.

Intense Contractions: The pain of contractions isn't necessarily greater during this transitional stage, but they are very close together and long, making them feel incredibly intense.

Empty Bladder and Consistent Nourishment: Ensure you empty your bladder approximately every hour and maintain consistent fluid intake. This keeps you hydrated and also makes room for your baby to descend.

Active Labor: Emotionally

The emotional landscape during active labor can feel as intense as the contractions themselves. Here's what you might experience:

Mixed Feelings: In the early part of active labor, you may wrestle with mixed feelings of excitement and anxiety. The anticipation of meeting your baby is intertwined with the uncertainty and some self-doubt may emerge.

Intensifying Contractions: As contractions intensify, you may encounter a range of emotions, including moments of worry, doubt, and surprise at the intensity and pain.

Loss of Control: You might struggle to feel 'in control' as you realize that labor is a force of nature, not something within your control. As you feel a sense of losing control, it's the perfect opportunity to choose to surrender to the process of labor.

Release and Surrender: If you feel safe and supported, you'll likely relinquish control and surrender to the labor process, embracing the powerful force of your body.

Tears and Overwhelm: It's entirely common to experience tears of overwhelm, fear, and uncertainty. These emotions are a natural response to the profound sensations and changes your body is undergoing.

Focus and Engagement: Despite the emotional fluctuations, you'll remain focused and engaged as contractions rhythmically persist.

Tuning Out Distractions: You may become easily annoyed or overwhelmed by distractions. Extra noise or activity can be overstimulating during this intense phase. Having a quiet and calm environment may be preferred and requested.

Fear and Frustration: As contractions get stronger, longer, and closer, you might experience moments of fear, anger, and frustration, especially during the transition phase when your body is dilating from 8-10cm.

Support is Vital: You'll feel that the support and assistance of others are crucial during this stage. Rely on your support team to help you find your rhythm, stay anchored, and remain relaxed through and between contractions.

Transition to the Birthplace: By this stage, you might feel ready to transition from home to the birth center or hospital, an excellent sign that your labor is progressing.

Emotional Expression in Active Labor

The idea of communicating your feelings and thoughts as they emerge during active labor is a crucial aspect of ensuring a positive and efficient birthing experience. It's common to experience a wide range of emotions during this stage, including excitement, anxiety, doubt, and sometimes even fear. The intensity of contractions can be surprising and challenging, often surpassing expectations.

The Power of Expression

One valuable tools at your disposal during active labor is the act of expression. Communicating your emotions and thoughts as they emerge is a powerful way to navigate the journey more effectively. Here's why this practice is so crucial:

Emotional Release: Labor is a deeply emotional process. The act of giving voice to your feelings, whether they are positive or challenging, can provide an emotional release. It allows you to acknowledge and process your emotions in real-time, preventing them from building up and becoming overwhelming.

Reducing Tension: Emotions can be physicalized in the body as tension, which can hinder the progress of labor. By expressing your emotions, you release this tension, allowing your body to work more efficiently.

Emotional Support: Your birth support team, including your doula, partner, or midwife, is there to provide emotional support. Sharing your feelings with them allows them to tailor their support to your specific needs, offering reassurance, encouragement, or a listening ear.

Increased Comfort: Expression helps you feel more comfortable, both physically and emotionally, during the challenges of active labor. It's an empowering practice that reminds you that you have agency and a voice in your birthing experience. It also increases your sense of feeling safe and secure, pivotal emotions in being able to let go in labor.

Enhanced Communication: Effective communication with your birth support team ensures that you receive the support you need. If you're struggling with a particular aspect of labor, articulating your feelings allows your team to make adjustments, suggest coping techniques, and provide the care that is tailored to you and your specific needs in the moment.

Overcoming Fears and Doubts

In active labor, it's not uncommon to encounter moments of doubt, fear, or surprise. You might question your ability to continue or wonder how much longer you can endure the intensity. Expressing these feelings can be transformative. Sharing your thoughts and fears can be met with reassurance, encouragement, and reminders of your inner strength. It's a process of acknowledging the doubts and then letting them go, making space for the courage and determination needed to continue.

The Slowdown of Holding In Emotions

Conversely, holding in your emotions can slow down or hinder the labor process. Emotions, especially fear and tension, can manifest as physical resistance in your body. This resistance can interfere with the natural progression of labor and the effectiveness of contractions. By expressing your emotions, you allow your body to respond in a more relaxed and productive manner.

Communicating your feelings and thoughts as they arise during active labor is an invaluable coping technique and tool for both your emotional well-being and the efficiency of the birthing process. It's a way to release tension, seek emotional support, and foster a sense of control and empowerment. Sharing your emotions is a vital part of ensuring a positive birthing experience.

Active Labor: Your Support Team

Leaning on your support team during active labor will help even the most intense moments of labor feel more manageable. Having a trusted and supportive team can really make the biggest difference in your birth experience during active labor. Here's are some very practical and specific ways your support team can come alongside you during active labor:

Practical Support

Time Contractions: Periodically time your contractions, observing you and noting any significant changes in behavior or frequency of contractions.

Contact Provider: Communicate with your healthcare provider to keep them updated on your progress or letting them know you are in labor.

Offer Food and Drink: Remind you to eat and drink and offer you water and small snacks frequently to help you maintain your energy levels.

Bathroom Breaks: Encourage you to use the bathroom every hour or so, ensuring your comfort and helping maintain the most room for baby to descend.

Emotional Support

Undivided Attention: Offer very focused and intentional attention; focus on your needs and support you as you transition through your rhythms.

Reassurance and Encouragement: Offer you the much needed reassurance and encouragement. Provide affirmations and a sense of confidence in you and the birth process.

Calm Presence: Stay connected through eye contact, steady touch and a calm, quiet voice, ensuring you feel grounded and supported.

Emotional Expression: Encourage you to express your emotions freely. Sometimes, just the act of sharing your feelings can provide significant relief.

Help with Rhythms

Anchor in Rhythm: Remind you of the importance of your chosen rhythm as an essential anchor through active labor.

Comfort Measures: Suggest comfort measures and coping techniques to ease the intensity of contractions.

Position Changes: Observe your movements and assist in guiding you through position changes every 5-10 contractions for optimal comfort.

Steady Touch: Intentional and steady touch, including counter pressure, acupressure, and massage, can be highly beneficial.

No Questions During Contractions: Avoid asking questions during contractions and stick to simple yes/no inquiries.

Medication Choices: Respect your autonomy and allow you to request pain medications when you feel it's necessary.

Active Labor: Coping Techniques

Coping Techniques in active labor will help you engage your whole self - body, mind, heart - allowing for a beautiful synchronicity that will feel so empowering.

Finding Your Rhythm

When you find your rhythm during active labor, you establish a comforting and grounding routine. This rhythm is a carefully selected combination of coping techniques that resonate with you. It becomes your trusted companion, offering a sense of predictability and control amidst the unpredictability of labor.

As a contraction approaches, you instinctively shift into your chosen rhythm. This sequence of coping techniques acts as an anchor, helping you prepare for the upcoming surge of energy. It allows you to focus your attention and energy where it is most needed, directing your mind and body toward the strength you need to work through each contraction.

The Flow Through Contractions

As the contraction intensifies and reaches its peak, your rhythm becomes your lifeline. It serves as a guide, allowing you to navigate the wave of intensity with an openness and calm surrender. You ride the wave, breathing through it, vocalizing if it helps, and finding a flow that enables you to navigate the sensation.

By staying in your rhythm, you establish a sense of calm within the strong waves of active labor. This rhythm becomes an oasis in the midst of powerful surges. It helps you open both physically and emotionally, allowing your body to progress through labor with greater ease.

Relaxation Between Contractions

Crucially, your rhythm isn't only about managing contractions but also about providing comfort and relaxation between them. In those brief moments of respite, you can rest and rejuvenate. Your body and mind get a chance to recover and prepare for the next contraction. It's a pause in the symphony of labor, allowing you to gather your strength and focus.

The Power of Change

Now, here's where the beauty of change comes into play. Change is not only inevitable in labor; it's also highly beneficial. It's a dynamic force that can propel you forward. By changing your rhythm every 5-10 contractions, you introduce variety and adaptability into your labor experience.

In essence, the concept of finding and changing rhythms during active labor empowers you to navigate this transformative stage with intention and adaptability. It's the art of balancing continuity with fluidity, ensuring that you have a steady anchor while being open to the shifts and changes that occur naturally in the birthing process. Rhythms help you stay present to the essence of active labor, where strength, rhythm, and change harmonize to guide you.

Choosing the coping techniques that make up your rhythms before labor will serve you so well. You will have a plethora of options to pull from in the midst of labor. Here is a list of coping techniques to explore and start using during pregnancy. The more coping techniques you have implored during pregnancy the more options you have to choose from when creating your rhythms. Pick 3-5 coping techniques that are your core techniques that you can naturally default to in the most intense moments of labor.

During active labor, it's essential to engage your entire self to navigate the intensity with strength and resilience. Your body, mind, and heart all play vital roles in creating a rhythm that will carry you through beautifully. Let's take a close look into the various rhythmic techniques and their practical applications during labor:

Rhythmic Movement

Sway and Rock: Gently swaying and rocking can mimic the soothing motion of the womb, promoting relaxation and comfort. It also creates more dynamic space in your pelvis making room for baby to move down and through. These movements can be done standing, sitting, or while kneeling, depending on what feels most natural to you at the time.

Squatting: Squatting is a powerful position to encourage your baby's descent and relieve pressure on your back. Your doula or partner can support you in maintaining this posture during contractions.

Hip Shaking: Partner involvement can be incredibly reassuring. Your partner can gently shake your hips to ease tension in the pelvic area, providing you with a calming, rhythmic touch.

Toilet Sitting: Sitting forward or backward on the toilet, using a stool or block to create asymmetry, can aid in progressing labor. The alternating elevation of one foot can be especially helpful in creating space for baby to descend.

Birth Ball Movements: Sitting on a birth ball, moving in circular or figure-eight motions, or engaging in gentle bouncing can provide both physical support and rhythmic comfort during contractions.

Hands and Knees: Adopting the yoga cat/cow pose or simply getting on your hands and knees can create a soothing rhythm, allowing you to focus on your breath and be in tone with your body.

Pelvic Rock: This movement, whether performed with knees bent or in a hands-and-knees position, helps open the pelvic area and promote baby's descent.

Walking/Pacing: Walking back and forth, whether in your birthing space or outside if possible, allows you to maintain a rhythmic pace and stay mobile.

Chair/Stool Use: Alternating elevated open leg positions using a chair or stool can relieve discomfort and introduce a rhythmic element to your movements.

Dangling: Leaning backward or forward on your partner during contractions can provide both emotional support and a comfort.

Slow Dance: Swaying back and forth with your arms around your partner's neck can create an intimate, rhythmic connection and offer some rest during labor.

Thumb Sucking (Lollipops): Sucking on a lollipop can be a comforting and rhythmic way to capture your senses and provide distraction from discomfort.

Lift and Tuck: Abdominal lifting, with partner support against a wall, is a technique that promotes optimal fetal positioning. [For detailed instructions on Lift and Tuck, visit: https://www.spinningbabies.com/pregnancy-birth/techniques/abdominal-lift-tuck]

Shower and Bath: Water is known for its calming effects, and taking a warm shower or bath can allow for your relaxation to go to a whole other level.

Standing with Head Resting: Placing your head on a table, bed, birth ball, peanut ball, or support of pillows, creates a comfortable and rhythmic rest position.

Exaggerated Side-Lying: Laying on your side with a pillow or peanut ball between your legs helps encourage rest while keeping a dynamic position in your pelvis.

Rhythmic Sounds

Diaphragmatic Breathing: Deep, diaphragmatic breathing, also known as "belly breathing," accompanied by humming or singing, can help you stay centered and rhythmic in your breath.

Vocalization: Experiment with low, deep vocalizations and moaning to express and release tension during contractions. Going deep and low encourages you to relax and open your pelvic floor muscles which allows for dilation.

Blowing Air: Gently blowing air out through your mouth, or making horse-like lips, can create a soothing and rhythmic breathing pattern.

Affirmations: Repeating positive and affirming phrases, either out loud or in your mind, offers a rhythmic mantra to focus on throughout each contraction. Your partner or doula can also read affirmations between contractions to maintain a supportive rhythm.

Mouth and Jaw Relaxation: Keeping your mouth open and relaxed, with or without sound, can aid in dissipating tension and encourages dilation.

Music: Immersing yourself in your chosen music can create a rhythmic backdrop to your labor, helping you stay grounded and focused.

Rhythmic Thoughts

Visualization: Envision the expansion and opening of your body, welcoming your baby's descent as you ride the waves of labor.

Positive Memories: Recall cherished memories, engaging all five senses and infusing them with vibrant colors to help anchor your mind.

Imagery: Consider visualizing contractions as waves, watching them rise, peak, and gently subside. Enjoy the pause between the waves and let your body fully relax.

Focusing Techniques: Choose a focal point to fix your gaze upon during contractions, staying firmly rooted in the present moment. Remind yourself to take one contraction or one breath at a time to stay present and confident.

Rhythmic Breathing

Rhythmic Breathing and Moaning: Combining rhythmic breathing with moaning can help you relax and channel your energy effectively.

Slow Breathing/Moaning: A deep, cleansing breath with a big sigh or moan after each contraction encourages you to release any tension out of your body between contractions, that way you don't go into the next one holding tension from the one before.

Light Breathing: Breathing in short, light breaths through the mouth, accompanied by a silent in-breath, an audible out-breath, and a brief pause, can create a rhythmic breathing cycle of 30-60 breaths per minute. This method has become less popular then the deeper, fuller breath methods but some mom's natural lean on a breathing pattern of short, quick breaths.

Rhythmic Touch

Rubbing, Scratching, Tapping, and Stroking: These tactile sensations can provide a comforting and rhythmic presence during labor, helping to release tension and promote relaxation. Sometimes you do this yourself or your partner or doula may help with this rhythmic touch.

Counter Pressure: Whether applied to the lower back or hips, counter pressure can be an extremely helpful technique to alleviate discomfort. Using a massage ball or tennis ball against a wall, bed, or bathtub can also offer similar relief.

Double Hip Squeezes: This technique, performed by your birth support team, involves applying rhythmic pressure to your hips, offering relief and emotional connection.

Hot/Cold Compresses: The alternation between hot and cold compresses can create a soothing rhythm and help manage pain and release tension and help regulate temperature that often fluctuations in labor from extremes.

Massage: Focusing on areas of tension with rhythmic massage techniques can ease muscle discomfort and promote relaxation. Gentle strokes and massage in early labor and more firm, steady touch in active labor tends to be preferred for many moms.

Criss-Cross Massage: Applying criss-cross massage strokes over the small of your back can offer rhythmic relief during contractions.

Breaking the Popsicle: A rhythmic hand or foot massage can be deeply soothing during labor, allowing you to channel your focus and energy.

Acupressure: Ho-ku Point and Spleen 6: Applying firm pressure to these acupressure points can help relieve pain and discomfort during contractions, they are often used to help induce or nudge labor forward.

Encouraging Head-to-Toe Relaxation: Your support team can gently touch and name any tense body parts during contractions, reminding you to relax your jaw, hands, bottom, pelvis, and feet. This rhythmic approach to relaxation can foster a calm and empowered birthing experience, allowing you to focus on releasing tension in each area of your body.

This holistic approach engages your whole self—body, mind, and heart—during active labor, providing a multifaceted toolkit to cope with the intensity and empower you as you bring your baby into the world. By choosing from these techniques in each of these categories, and making small alterations to your rhythm every 5-10 contractions, you'll be well-prepared to embrace each contraction in labor.

4

Pushing: The Power of Your Body

As you move through the stages of labor, you will encounter a renewed wave of energy and a rush of hormones as you approach the pushing stage. This is the moment when you might feel like you've given it your all during early and active labor, and your energy reserves seem depleted. But fear not; nature has a way of providing you with the strength and vitality you need for this pivotal stage.

Pushing, will reveal to you how incredibly strong and capable you are and you will see the remarkable synergy between your body, mind, and heart. To make this stage as efficient and empowering as possible, it's essential to understand the options available and the techniques that can facilitate your pushing best.

Pushing Methods

Laboring Down

Before we dive into the two main styles of pushing, it's crucial to highlight the concept of "laboring down." Laboring down involves waiting until the urge to push becomes irresistibly strong, a sensation that is nearly impossible to resist. Initially, this urge may feel mild or brief at the peak of a contraction. If you have received an epidural, it's common to feel pressure that is increasing and persistent; adopting an upright seated position and allowing your baby to descend to a +2/+3 station before commencing the pushing phase is often referred to as laboring down.

Guided Pushing

One approach to pushing is guided pushing, in which a nurse, midwife, or obstetrician looks at the monitors or feels on your belly for the onset of a contraction and then guides you through the process. This guidance typically involves holding your breath, curling around your baby with your chin down, elbows out, and pulling your legs towards you while laying on your back (usually in stirrups) or on your side. You are encouraged to push three times in a row with each contraction, holding your breath and bearing down as intensely as possible.

Some providers may stretch the vaginal area and apply oil to minimize friction. Additionally, hot compresses can be used to reduce the risk of tearing. Guided pushing is particularly beneficial when you've had an epidural and might not have a clear sense of when a contraction is occurring or how to push effectively.

Self-Directed Pushing

Another style of pushing is self-directed pushing, which encourages you to listen to your body's cues. You'll pay attention as each contraction builds, and when it reaches its peak, you will bear down in response to your body's urging. Contractions during this stage can vary in length and strength, and you'll follow your body's lead. Utilizing diaphragmatic or glottis breathing techniques can be particularly helpful in self-directed pushing.

You will have the flexibility to move into positions that your body finds most comfortable for pushing. This might involve squatting, semi-squatting, hands and knees, or side-lying positions, among others. The primary goal during self-directed pushing is to follow your body's rhythm and use each contraction to its fullest potential.

Tips for Pushing

Regardless of the pushing style, there are several tips to keep in mind as you push:

Wait for it to build: Allow the urge or pressure to build to it's peak, find your full breath, and then bare down using the full strength and length of your contraction.

Keep hips wide and open OR knees together: You have the option to alternate between these positions as you push.

Push to your limit and beyond: Babies often make the most significant progress just beyond the point that feels like your limit.

Push towards the pressure: Your instinct may be to pull back or hold back as you feel the pressure and intensity that comes with the pushing stage. Directing your efforts towards the pressure sensation, focusing on going towards and with the pressure, will assist the baby's descent.

Find a rhythm: Just like in active labor, finding a rhythm encourages you to push most effectively. At first, you may feel uncertain about how effective you are or if your pushing is even working, that's normal. As baby continues to descend, the urge or pressure gets even stronger and you will instinctively find a rhythm. With an epidural, having some specific guidance at first is helpful but usually mom's start feeling the rhythm and pressure and start leading the way.

Embrace the unique sensations of pushing, and trust in your body's wisdom to bring your baby into the world. Your birth doula will typically be right by your side as you push, giving you tips and gentle reminders to guide you through the pushing stage. A doula helps you feel confident and capable in this very proactive stage where you are working intently with your body.

The moment your baby is in your arms is a culmination of indescribable emotions and an overwhelming rush of love, wonder, and awe. It's a profound fusion of vulnerability and strength, as you bring a new life into the world with your unwavering determination, strength and resolve. In that instant, the world narrows to the miracle and magic of this new existence, and a deep, timeless connection is forged, forever etching this extraordinary moment in your heart.

Breathing Techniques

During the pushing stage of labor, your choice of breathing techniques can impact the effectiveness of your pushing and the pace at which pushing moves. Let's explore two primary methods: holding your breath and diaphragmatic or glottis pushing, along with their pros and cons.

Holding Your Breath Pushing

Holding your breath during pushing is a common technique used in labor, especially if you have an epidural. It's the typical guidance you can anticipate receiving from your provider. Here's how to do it effectively:

Get in Position: Position yourself comfortably for pushing. This can vary depending on your preferences and the guidance of your healthcare provider. Common positions include lying on your back, sitting up, tug-of-war, squatting, or using a squat bar. Choose the position that feels most comfortable and effective for you. Changing position every 30 minutes or so is very helpful to create dynamic change in your pelvis and encourage baby to move through your birth canal.

Find the Right Time: Before you start holding your breath, it's important you time it with the peak of your contraction. You will typically feel a strong urge to push or a building pressure and your healthcare provider can help confirm that you are having a contraction.

Take a Deep Breath: Before a contraction begins, take a deep breath in through your nose. Inhale as deeply as you can to fill your lungs.

Hold Your Breath: As the contraction starts and you feel the urge to push, hold your breath. You can close your mouth and keep the air in your lungs.

Push with All Your Strength: During the contraction, push with all your strength while holding your breath. Focus on directing your energy toward pushing your baby downward. Push as if you're having a bowel movement. Your healthcare provider or nurse may instruct you to count to ten as you push.

Exhale Slowly: Once the contraction ends, exhale slowly and evenly through your mouth. This step is crucial to prevent a sudden drop in your blood oxygen levels.

Rest and Repeat: Between contractions, take a moment to rest and recover. You should be breathing normally and not holding your breath during these intervals. Take some full breaths in as you rest between contractions to provide yourself and your baby with optimal levels of oxygen. Contractions are typically spaced out, giving you time to recuperate between each effort.

Listen to Your Healthcare Provider: Follow the guidance of your healthcare provider or midwife. They will instruct you on when to start and stop pushing and ensure that you're using the holding-your-breath technique effectively.

Pros to Holding Your Breath Pushing:

- **Increased Intra-abdominal Pressure:** Holding your breath during pushing generates greater intra-abdominal pressure. This pressure can assist in effectively moving the baby through the birth canal by pushing against the cervix and guiding the baby downward.
- **Boosted Pushing Strength:** Holding your breath enables you to direct all your energy toward pushing. This can be particularly beneficial in helping you make the most of each contraction.

Cons to Holding Your Breathe Pushing:

- **Reduced Oxygen Supply:** One significant drawback is that holding your breath diminishes your oxygen supply. It can lead to a drop in your blood oxygen levels, which isn't ideal for you or the baby.
- **Increased Stress:** Holding your breath can increase stress levels. It can be a more intense and challenging experience, potentially leading to exhaustion and greater discomfort.

Diaphragmatic Breathing for Pushing

Diaphragmatic breathing, also known as "belly breathing," is a technique that focuses on deep, controlled breaths using your diaphragm muscle. This method is especially useful during labor as it ensures a consistent oxygen supply and helps you stay relaxed. Here's how to diaphragmatically breathe during labor and pushing:

Find a Comfortable Position: Begin by finding a comfortable position that supports deep breathing. You can sit or lie down on your side or back, whatever feels best for you.

Place Your Hand on Your Abdomen: To practice diaphragmatic breathing, you can start by placing one hand on your abdomen, just below your ribcage.

Inhale Slowly Through Your Nose: Inhale deeply and slowly through your nose. Focus on filling your abdomen with air rather than just your chest.

Exhale Gradually Through Your Mouth: Exhale slowly and evenly through your mouth. As you exhale, visualize the breath helping move your baby down and out.

Maintain a Steady Rhythm: Establish a consistent, steady rhythm for your breathing in both your inhalation and exhalation; adjust your breathing to align with the length and strength of your contraction.

Focus on Relaxation: As you breathe deeply, concentrate on baring down through the contraction.

Use This Technique During all of Labor: Using diaphragmatic breathing during labor will help you naturally defer to it during the pushing stage. It will help you stay relaxed and ensure a steady oxygen supply for you and your baby.

Glottis Breathing for Pushing

Glottis pushing involves making a low-pitched sound or closing your vocal cords to create resistance during the push. This technique can increase intra-abdominal pressure, which can be particularly useful during the pushing stage of labor. Here's how to use glottis pushing:

Find Your Voice: During a contraction, as you feel the urge to push, find your voice and make a low-pitched, guttural sound. This sound is similar to a deep, throaty growl or groan.

Close Your Vocal Cords: As you make the sound, consciously close your vocal cords. This action creates resistance, allowing you to push more effectively.

Push with the Sound: As you push with each contraction, use the low-pitched sound as a guide. It can help you push more efficiently while reducing the risk of holding your breath.

Breathe Normally Between Contractions: In between contractions, return to your regular breathing pattern. This ensures you're getting enough oxygen and helps prevent hyperventilation.

Listen to Your Body: Pay close attention to your body's cues. Push when you feel the strong urge during a contraction and use the glottal sound to guide your efforts.

Glottis pushing can help increase the effectiveness of your pushes.

Pros of Diaphragmatic or Glottis Pushing:

- **Sustained Oxygen Supply:** Diaphragmatic or glottis pushing involves controlled breathing techniques, which means you maintain a steady oxygen supply. This is crucial for both your well-being and the baby's.
- **Less Stress and Fatigue:** These techniques can lead to a less stressful and fatiguing pushing stage. You're able to maintain a sense of control and may experience less overall discomfort.
- **Reduced Risk of Hyperventilation:** With controlled breathing, you're less likely to hyperventilate, which can sometimes occur during breath-holding and lead to dizziness or lightheadedness.

Cons of Diaphragmatic or Glottis Pushing:

- **Potentially Slower Progress:** Diaphragmatic or glottis pushing may result in slower progress during the pushing stage. The reduced intra-abdominal pressure means you might not push as forcefully, potentially elongating the stage.
- **Increased Perceived Pain:** Some individuals find that controlled breathing techniques lead to an increased perception of pain. While this may be due to the slower progress, it's important to be aware that discomfort can be more pronounced.

The choice between holding your breath and using diaphragmatic or glottis pushing depends on your personal preferences, comfort level, and the specific circumstances of your labor. It's important to discuss these options with your healthcare provider and birth support team in advance so that you can make an informed decision when the time comes. Trying multiple ways to breathe (both prenatally and in the moment) to discover which method works best for you. Additionally, be open to adjustments during labor if your chosen technique isn't providing the desired results, as flexibility can be essential in ensuring a successful and comfortable birth.

Pushing with an Epidural

In the lead-up to the pushing stage with an epidural, you'll often feel a mix of sensations and emotions. While the epidural provides pain relief, you may still experience some discomfort, particularly as the contractions intensify in the transition stage (8cm-10cm dilation). There's typically a surge of hormones and adrenaline, creating a sense of restlessness and unease. You'll start feeling excitement for meeting your baby and an eagerness, strength, and motivation for pushing. Nausea might also be present, along with a feeling of anticipation. These sensations are often signs that pushing is imminent.

If you've had a very long and tiring labor or induction, it's not uncommon to feel worried or uncertain as pushing is approaching. Mainly wondering "will I have the energy and strength to push feeling this tired, hungry and weak." Many mom's don't eat once they have their epidural placed which adds an additional layer of depletion. Rest assured, you will have what you need to push your baby. Even the most tired mom finds the energy and momentum she needs to push. A big part of that surge of motivation and confidence is dependent on your support team, the extra encouragement and guidance for pushing gives you the extra energy you need to give it all you've got.

During the pushing stage with an epidural, sensations can be quite different from an unmedicated labor. You might feel a pressure and stretching sensation as the baby's head descends through the birth canal.

While you may not experience pain, you often feel the intensity of the moment and the effort required to push effectively. Many mom's describe it as the biggest workout of their life. The support of a birthing team, including your birth doula, becomes crucial during this phase, as you may be more reliant on guidance and encouragement to push effectively. When the baby is crowning, there's a unique combination of pressure and a stretching sensation, which can be uncomfortable but not typically painful due to the epidural. It's a moment filled with anticipation and excitement as the baby's arrival becomes imminent. Receiving emotional support, coaching, and reassurance is essential as the pushing process unfolds.

Pushing Stage of Labor

Let's unravel the physical, emotional, and the vital role of your support team during the pushing stage of labor. This is a crucial juncture where the power of your body, the focus of your mind, and the courage of your heart converge to bring your baby into the world. As a birth doula, I hope with this guidance, encouragement, and support you will navigate pushing with confidence, courage and the knowledge that you alone have what it takes to birth your baby and that you are not alone in this beautiful process.

Pushing: Physically

The pushing stage of labor is a uniquely individual journey, with its length varying from one mother to another and from one pregnancy to the next.

It can span anywhere from just a few contractions to lasting several hours. Before and during pushing, contractions might space out, granting you a momentary break and a chance to rest, although this doesn't occur in every labor. Transition contractions are typically 1-2 minutes apart and feel right on top of each other, just before you start pushing and while pushing you may get back to 3-5 minute apart contractions.

You'll likely experience surges of the oxytocin hormone, which create a potent urge and uncontrollable sensation to push.

Your baby will rotate and descend, with part of baby's head becoming visible at the vaginal opening. This stage can be a rhythmic dance as the baby rocks back and forth with contractions until the head progresses past the pubic bone.

It's also important to support the perineum and use warm compresses, as they can help reduce the likelihood of tearing.

Once your baby is born, you'll have a brief respite before feeling contractions again, and you'll experience the urge to push once more, this time to deliver the placenta.

Your provider will check for bleeding levels and make any necessary repairs to the perineum shortly after the placenta is delivered.

Fundal massage to assess the firmness of the uterus and a check along with repairs for tears often come with a reasonable amount of discomfort.

Pushing: Emotionally

You'll likely feel relief and excitement upon reaching full dilation, with renewed energy propelling you forward. There's a newfound enthusiasm and motivation to push and bring your baby into the world.

An uncontrollable surge of desire to push will wash over you, although you might initially feel uncertain about the right technique. Questions like, "Is this working?" and "Is this how I should push?" may cross your mind until you get into you find your rhythm in pushing.

You might also experience a natural instinct to hold back or pull away as you sense the pressure in the vagina, perhaps accompanied by a touch of fear or alarm.

The act of pushing can feel rewarding, empowering, and filled with determination for some, while others may find it tough, painful, and exhausting.

The "Ring of Fire" sensation, as your baby crowns, brings about a strong burning, stinging, and pressure.

Once your baby emerges, emotions of excitement, joy, empowerment, and even shock may take hold.

Be prepared for some discomfort or pain during postpartum procedures such as fundal massages, vaginal checks and repairs for tears.

Pushing: Your Support Team

Your support team places a significant role during your pushing stage; it can really feel like a team. Though you are doing all the physical work, your support team's encouragement and guidance is pivotal.

Your support will inquire about your pushing preferences and assist you in finding different positions that work for you.

Helpful hands on support such as encouraging words, being at your side, setting the environment (music, lighting, aromatherapy) and providing a cold compress for your face or neck as the exertion of pushing might make you feel warm will feel so welcomed.

Supporting your position, holding a leg, or offering a resting spot between pushes are all part of your support team's role.

Reminding you of pushing tips, ensuring you're well-prepared and adjusting as you seek to find the most effective ways to push.

After your baby is born, caring for your needs are so important, making sure you are warm and comfortable with a cozy blanket, particularly if you're experiencing any shaking.

Your support team should be well-versed in newborn procedure preferences and your personal choices to communicate with the providers when you might be focused on pushing or immediate postpartum care.

Hydration and nourishment are essential, so your support should make sure to offer food and drink shortly after birth, per provider indication.

Pushing: Coping Techniques

In the throes of the pushing stage, a mosaic of techniques and sensations comes into play, guided by the rhythm of your labor and the innate wisdom of your body. Here are some essential strategies to consider:

Change positions every 30 minutes or 5-10 contractions: Shifting your posture is not only about comfort but also encouraging your baby's descent.

Take several deep breaths: Deep, cleansing breaths allow you to center yourself, gather strength, provide oxygen to you and your baby and focus your energy where it's needed most.

Breathe through pushing: Despite the powerful urge to push, controlled breathing helps maintain your rhythm and energy.

Let your body guide when to push: Your body has an internal rhythm that syncs with your baby's descent. Let it lead the way.

Push with your contractions: Trust your body's cues. Pushing should be purposeful but not forced, guided by your instincts and the rhythm of contractions.

Wait for the contraction to build and peak: As the contraction intensifies, bear down with it, using its natural momentum to your advantage.

Bear down and relax pelvic floor simultaneously: These movements work in harmony to pave the way for your baby's descent.

Push towards, not away from, the pressure and pain: Counter intuitive as it may seem, directing your efforts toward the source of pressure can facilitate progress.

Push beyond your limit: When you feel like you've reached your limit with a push, give an extra effort to push beyond what feels like your limit. Often times, that last strong and focused effort at the end of a push can make a big difference in moving baby down and past the pubic bone.

Chin down, back arched: These postural adjustments optimize the space in your pelvis and birth canal creating more room for baby to come through.

Squeeze hips to help the baby move down: Gentle pressure on the hips can create space and support your baby's descent.

Rest between contractions: These brief interludes provide a chance to recuperate, recharge, and gather your strength.

Knees up and elbows out: This position can be particularly effective in opening up the pelvis, providing a balance between stability and openness.

Knees together: Sometimes, closing the gap can be as important as opening it, creating dynamic space in your pelvis.

Tug of war: Involving your partner by handing them a sheet can create a sense of teamwork and shared effort. It adds an extra layer of connection during this profound moment. It also allows for you to use your force and curl around your belly effectively.

Slow or stop pushing during crowning: When your baby is on the cusp of crowning, a controlled approach, such as slowing down or panting, can minimize tearing, allowing the contraction to assist in the final force that allows baby to be born.

Position Options for Pushing Stage

During the pushing stage, the positions you choose can significantly impact your comfort, the progress of your labor, and your baby's descent. During pushing, explore these positions, seek to find the ones that align best with your preferences and needs. It's likely you will change positions several times (especially a first time mom) so don't feel stuck to just the one you start with:

Side Lying: This position offers a relaxed, horizontal stance. It's particularly useful for conserving energy and allowing your body to focus entirely on pushing. It's often a welcome choice after an intense active labor.

Squatting/Supported Squat: Squatting provides the advantage of gravity, aiding your baby's descent. Whether using a squat bar or the support of your partner, this position can be empowering. Supported squatting eases the strain on your legs and is ideal for conserving energy.

Hands and Knees: Assuming a hands-and-knees position can alleviate pressure on your back, providing relief from the intensity of contractions. This posture also encourages your baby to maneuver more easily into the birth canal.

Asymmetrical Kneeling: Kneeling with one leg raised or extended provides variety and flexibility. It can be helpful in promoting your baby's optimal positioning for birth.

Lunge: The lunge position combines stretching with gravity's assistance. By allowing one leg to extend forward while the other remains bent, it can be an excellent choice for helping your baby navigate the pelvis.

Kneeling while leaning against an upright bed: This position takes advantage of the support the bed offers. You can find comfort and balance while focusing on the crucial work of pushing.

Birth Pool: Submerging yourself in a warm birth pool can be a soothing and pain-relieving option. The buoyancy supports your body, and the warm water helps relax your muscles and your perineum. It's not only conducive to pushing but also provides a serene, gentle and intimate setting for the birth of your baby.

Birth Stool/Toilet (at the start of pushing): The birth stool or a toilet can be an excellent choice as you transition into the pushing stage. These positions take advantage of the natural incline and gravity, aiding your baby's descent.

Back: This is the most recommended and typical choice in a hospital setting, especially if you have an epidural. This position is often suggested for medical interventions or specific clinical reasons. Depending on your provider team you may need to advocate for trying different positions other than laying on your back in stirrups.

Each of these positions serves a unique purpose, and their suitability may depend on your personal comfort and the dynamics of your labor.

Your provider and support team can help you explore and determine which position aligns best with your needs and the progress of your labor.

Engaging in a meaningful dialogue with your healthcare provider about your preferences for the pushing stage, including the various positions you'd like to explore, is a crucial step in your birth journey. Crafting a comprehensive birth plan that clearly outlines your position preferences empowers you to effectively communicate with every member of your support team when the day of labor arrives. This open communication ensures that your birthing experience aligns with your wishes and comfort, fostering a harmonious and supportive environment.

5

Turning Your Birth Vision Into Reality

We've spent time walking through each stage of labor and what you can anticipate – physically, emotionally, and mentally in an effort to help you feel prepared and equipped for labor. Now it's time to get really practical and start taking some intentional steps to achieving the birth you desire and deserve. Empowering yourself with personalized coping rhythms and affirmations can make a significant difference in your birthing experience. This purposeful preparation will give you the tools you need in your toolkit, helping you navigate each step of your labor with confidence and strength.

In this section, we'll explore two powerful strategies to enhance your readiness: creating personalized rhythms and crafting affirmations that resonate with your vision and address your preferences and concerns.

The preparation you'll do now will serve as valuable resources during labor and also contribute to a more positive and empowered pregnancy and help usher you into parenthood with confidence.

#1 Create Personalized Rhythms

One of the key preparations for labor is to create personalized rhythms that will serve as your anchors throughout the birthing process.

Using the coping techniques discussed in the previous chapters:

Step 1: Bundle 2-4 of them to form a rhythm bundle.

Step 2: Develop a list of at least 6-8 rhythms for each stage of labor.

Step 3: Walk through your home (together with your partner) and identify positions and activities you can engage in before heading to your birthing place. This will be a particularly beneficial strategy for early and early active labor.

Step 4: Select 2-3 coping techniques that deeply resonate with your body, mind, and heart on an emotional level. Pick 1 or 2 for your body, 1 or 2 for your mind, and 1 or 2 for heart (emotionally). These will be your core anchoring coping techniques, they will probably be part of each of your rhythms as you move and change positions.

Write down your core coping techniques and your rhythm bundles and share them with your support team so they can help remind you of your coping anchors during labor. It's crucial to practice these coping anchors during pregnancy to seamlessly integrate them into your birthing journey.

The goal is to practice them prenatally so that they become habitual and will naturally be your default in labor, even in the most intense moments of labor. Practice them when you experience discomfort or stress, allowing you to harness their power with ease.

#2 Create Personalized Affirmations

Deep within our minds, we each possess an internal reel of thoughts, often on a constant loop. These thoughts, stemming from our beliefs, experiences, and emotions, play a significant role in shaping our perspective and, in turn, our actions. Affirmations serve as powerful tools, allowing us to bring to the forefront of our consciousness the narratives we are playing in our minds. By becoming acutely aware of these thought reels, we gain the ability to intentionally choose the stories we tell ourselves, ultimately influencing the way we perceive the world and the actions we take, which in turn, molds our unique life experiences. It's a reminder that the power to shape our reality begins with the stories we weave within our own minds.

This exercise is an invitation into shaping the type of story you want to envision for your birth and being a proactive participant in making that a reality.

Step 1: Together with your partner, sit down and each individually write down your vision, desires, wishes, and preferences for your birth experience. Be explicit and consider how you want to *feel* throughout this process, as the emotional aspect is a vital component of creating your vision. Often, the feelings we envision can be maintained regardless of the specific details of labor.

Step 2: Individually list any fears, concerns, and worries you have regarding birth. Be specific, considering your own concerns, those related to your baby, and those affecting your partner.

Step 3: Using your vision, desires, and wishes, along with your fears, concerns, and worries, craft specific affirmations.

Affirmations are positively framed statements or phrases that reflect what you want to be true, even if they don't feel true at the moment. Repeating and reflecting on these affirmations throughout pregnancy increases the likelihood that they will align with your experience in pregnancy, birth, and postpartum.

Step 4: Once you've created your affirmations, find ways to incorporate them into your daily life. Write them on note cards, place them on your wall or mirror, or keep them readily accessible on your phone. Begin and end your day by repeating a few of your core affirmations, allowing them to guide your thoughts and feelings throughout your journey to motherhood.

Affirmations

Here are a list of affirmations that families have connected to and have found helpful in pregnancy, labor, & postpartum to help inspire you as you create your own. You might find that using some of these along with creating some of your own personalized ones will be just the right combination of affirmations for you.

My baby is strong and healthy.
  I trust my body.
  I am a strong and capable woman.
  I have patience.
  There is no need for us to hurry.

I am strong, calm and beautiful.
Birth is a wonderful, safe experience.
I ask my Higher Power for and receive what I need.
My baby is healthy.
I am surrounded by loving, nurturing support.
I fearlessly surrender
My body is nourishing my baby perfectly.
Birth comes easily to me.
I am whole and at peace.
I am aware of my balanced, calm center.
My body knows how to birth my baby.
I have everything I need.
My body is strong and flexible.
I cooperate with my body and my baby.
My baby knows how to be born.
I put all fear aside as I prepare for the birth of my baby.
Untapped sources of strength are available to me.
I am relaxed and happy
I am focused on a smooth, easy birth.
I trust my body to know what it is to do.
I welcome my coming labor as the perfect one for me and my baby.
My mind is relaxed, my body is relaxed.
I am an active and powerful woman.
I feel confident; I feel safe; I feel secure.
I welcome this opportunity to grow and change.
My muscles work in complete harmony to make birthing easier.
I relax as we move through each stage of birth.
My baby is in the perfect position for birth.
My cervix opens outward and allows my baby to ease down.
I fully relax and turn my birthing over to God.
I see my baby coming smoothly from my womb.

My baby's birth will be easy because I am so relaxed.
My breath is easy, deep, and full.
My baby will be born at the perfect moment.
My body knows exactly what to do.
Each surge of my body brings my baby closer to me.
My body is wise and purposeful.
I am totally relaxed and at ease.
I can handle whatever comes up.
My body remains still and completely relaxed.
I trust my intuition.
My baby is safe.
I put all fear aside and welcome my baby
with happiness and joy.
I am a wonderful mother.

6

Visuals for Labor Positions

Labor Positions

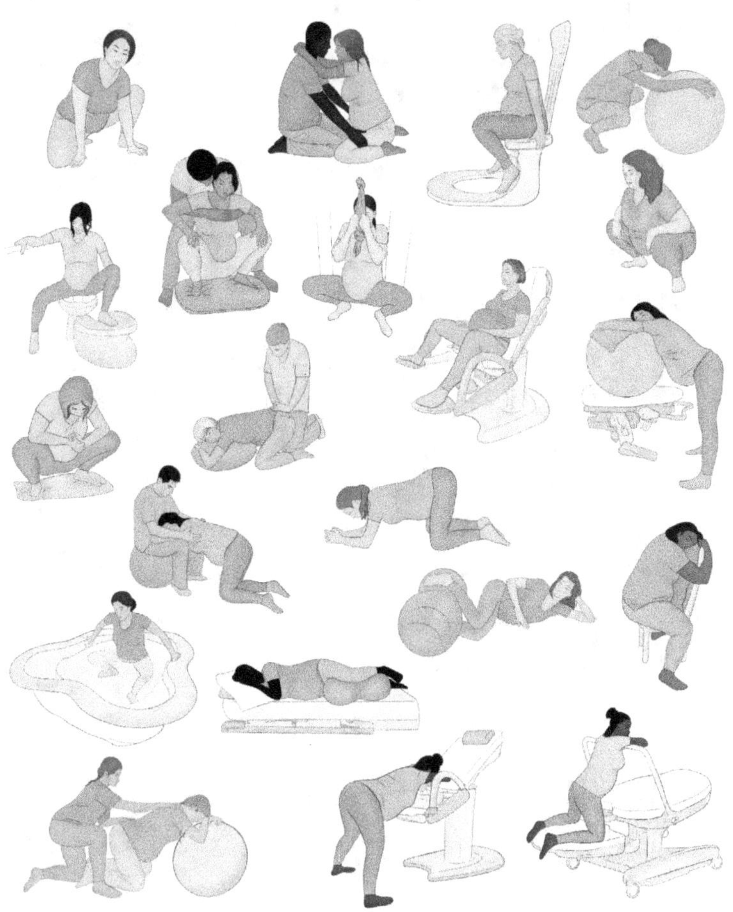

Positions for Pushing

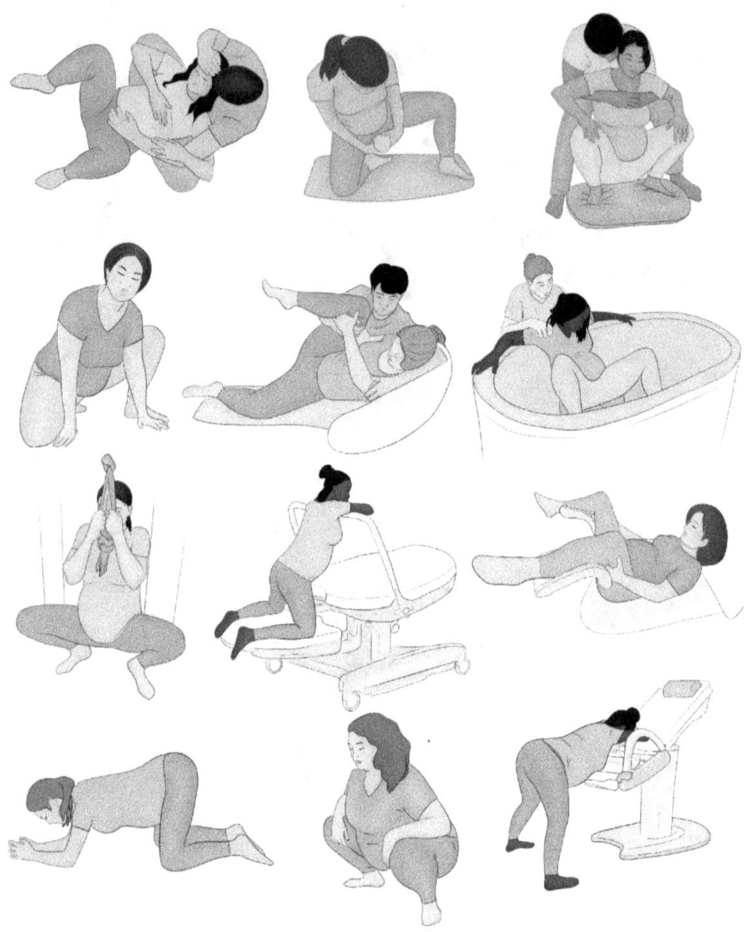

7

Do I Need Coping Techniques If I Get An Epidural?

Whether you are pursuing an unmedicated birth or know you want an epidural you will greatly benefit from understanding, practicing, and planning to use coping rhythms in labor. It will impact your birth in such profoundly positive ways.

Rhythms in labor, even after receiving an epidural, hold immense value in ensuring a positive and smooth birthing experience. While the epidural offers pain relief, it's so helpful to continue to mimic the physiological aspects of labor as closely as possible. This involves frequent and intentional position changes, which play a significant role in shortening the duration of labor and promoting the descent of your baby and proper alignment of your baby in the pelvis.

The epidural is one of the tools in your coping toolkit. When the rhythmic and dynamic strategies you've employed to manage labor reach their limit, it's a suitable moment to contemplate the use of an epidural. Even if you've already planned for an epidural at some stage during labor, it's highly beneficial to utilize coping techniques before its administration. These techniques not only complement your pain management plan but also enhance your overall birthing experience.

As a birth doula, I help moms change positions every thirty minutes once they have an epidural. Utilizing techniques such as Spinning Babies and the use of a peanut ball, stirrups, and pillows to help create variability and encourage the dynamic movement of the pelvis to make room for baby to descend. Position changes maintain your rhythm and keep labor progressing smoothly. This may involve shifting from side to side, using various sitting positions, or even adjusting the bed to an upright posture. You can even get onto hands and knees or squatting positions for labor and pushing with an epidural (depending on the denseness of the epidural and your mobility with it). These strategies can provide the comfort and support necessary for a positive experience, ultimately aiding the baby's descent and ensuring a smoother journey through the final stages of labor.

When's the best or right time for an epidural?

Timing when to get an epidural during labor is a highly individual decision, and the choice of when it is right for you is ultimately yours to make. There are pros and cons to consider, whether you opt for it earlier in labor or wait until labor is more active.

Getting an epidural early can provide relief from pain and allow you to rest if you've had a particularly challenging or long early labor. On the flip side, waiting until labor is more active can offer the advantage of a smoother transition into the pushing stage, which might lead to a shorter overall labor duration. When you choose an epidural in active labor (5-6cm dilated) the chance for labor to stop or stale becomes less likely, which means less intervention or need for augmentation of labor.

As a doula, I often suggest waiting until you feel that the pain has shifted from something you can manage to something more akin to suffering. This is often a good gauge to help you decide when the time is right for you and your unique labor experience.

By dedicating time during your prenatal preparation to explore and practice various coping techniques and rhythmic approaches for labor, you'll discover that managing early labor becomes something you can do with confidence and ease. Additionally, you'll acquire the skills to navigate even the most intense contractions, allowing you to stay within the discomfort and pain zone rather than crossing into a realm of suffering. This preparation will empower you when deciding on an epidural because it will feel like an additional tool or coping technique, rather than a desperate need to escape unbearable sensations or regain a sense of control that may have seemed lost.

Managing the emotional and mental aspects of labor can be a profound journey, particularly when you've initially planned for an unmedicated birth but opt for an epidural at some point in labor. It's entirely normal to experience a range of emotions during this transition. Some may feel a sense of disappointment or frustration, while others might find relief and empowerment in their choice. As a birth doula, I've witnessed many mothers navigate this shift with grace and courage. In fact, most of the mom's I support often feel a sense of pride for the strength and power it took to get through labor until the moment they choose an epidural.

Remember that childbirth is a dynamic experience, and your choices should always align with what feels like the right choice for you at that moment. Embrace the flexibility and adaptability that come with childbirth, knowing that the ultimate goal is a safe and positive birthing experience for both you and your baby, regardless of the path it takes.

Will I miss my chance to get an epidural if i wait too long?

No, not typically. Many mom's worry that if they wait to long they will miss their window in which an epidural can be placed. While at times labor does move very fast and a baby is born before a mom can get an epidural, in most cases, you can choose an epidural at any stage or point in labor that you want.

As a birth doula, I've seen mom's choose an epidural even when they were already 10cm dilated and ready to push. There isn't typically a 'to late' or a specific time window you have to be within if you want an epidural. Staying still while they place the epidural can be a little harder in a more active labor pattern, but mom's manage to stand still for the brief time they need to and anesthesiologists are great about waiting to place the epidural in-between contractions.

Different hospitals have different policies and capacities; it is worth having a conversation with your provider or asking during a hospital tour what the anesthesiologists at that given hospital are willing and able to do. Also, nurses in every setting have different approaches and recommendations. Sometimes nurses are eager to encourage and recommend an epidural and they recommend one early and often. Putting a request in your birth plan that states "allow me to ask for an epidural or pain management when I'm ready" will help reduce the chance that a nurse or provider will ask you about getting an epidural before you feel ready for one.

Ultimately, make your choice for an epidural more on what you need and want than on trying to time in 'just right' or letting the fear of not timing it right dictate your decision. With your birth rhythms for coping on hand, I trust you will navigate your labor leading up to an epidural with confidence and courage.

8

When Should I Go to the Hospital?

The question "When should I go to the hospital or birth center?" is often pressing for families. It's typically linked to fears like these: "What if I wait to long and my baby is born on the car ride?" or "What if I get there too late and I miss the chance to get my epidural?" or "What if I get there too early and I have to go back home?"

Knowing when the 'time is right' to go to the hospital can feel overwhelming. On the one hand you don't want to get there too early and either be at the hospital for many grueling hours/days or be encouraged to go back home. On the other hand, you don't want to feel so rushed or worried that you won't make it to the hospital in time – and have your baby in route. Finding the sweet spot for when to go to your birth place is different for each person based on their specific wishes and preferences for their birth. A birth doula can be a huge help in guiding you in making that decision for yourself in the heat of labor.

Here are a few tips or recommendations that can help you decide that it's time to go to your birth place:

3-1-1

Contractions are three minutes apart, last a minute long, and have been at this pace for at least an hour. The strength and length of the contraction are what you are looking for; contractions that are strong and long are the ones that usually make change to your cervix. So, if you are having 2-3 minute contractions but they are only 30-40 seconds long and mild, you may still be in the early stages of labor. Often, especially a first time mom, will head to their place of birth too soon. Choosing/changing rhythms will help you avoid leaving home earlier than needed. If this is a consecutive birth you might want to consider heading over at (5-1-1 or 4-1-1).

Anal Pressure

You begin to feel pressure in your anus. You may start to feel this pressure at the peak of a contraction and then it goes away between contractions. This pressure will continue to grow in intensity and duration. If you are feeling it throughout a contraction or even in between contractions you should head to your place of birth or contact your midwife team to come to your home. For the majority of your time at home you should not anticipate feeling anal pressure. If you are planning to get to the hospital in early active labor you will not feel this pressure while at home. This pressure emerges as baby descends lower and as your cervix becomes more and more dilated. You can trust you're in very active labor once you feel the anal pressure.

Tub Test

If your contractions are feeling strong, long and steady but you're not feeling quite ready to go to your birth place, try the Tub Test. Draw a bath (or a shower if a bath is not available). The bath often can relax your body and space out your contractions, especially if you are still in early active labor. It can also give you the extra relaxation and calm you need to feel like you can still comfortably manage at home. If you get in the bath and contractions continue to stay strong, long, and steady then it may be the sign you need to head to your birth space.

Please note that these recommendations are based on a mom who's preference is to stay home as long as possible. If that is not your goal, you would probably find it helpful to head to the hospital when contraction patterns are 5-1-1 or 4-1-1. You wont be waiting to for the sensation of anal pressure. Using the tub before going may be a nice option regardless, it can soothe your nerves, calm your mind, and ease the intensity of contractions making for a more gentle transition from home to the hospital or birth center.

As a birth doula, I can observe (if I'm in person) or hear (if I'm over the phone) when I mom has shifted into a more active labor pattern, the intensity that comes with that shift is very clear. Waiting for that shift within yourself, and staying present to observe it, can be a very helpful guide. Typically that shift comes with an acknowledgment and awareness that "this contractions are different or feel different"

9

75

How Can I Prevent Tearing While Pushing?

"I really don't want to tear" is often on the top three list for mom's when I ask them what they hope for in labor. Tearing during pushing is often one of the top three fears mom's express prenatally. Nobody wants to tear, it sounds awful, can be painful, and can impact your recovery postpartum. So, can it be avoided? And how?

Tearing during labor is a big worry for many moms-to-be, and it's something that's often on their minds throughout pregnancy and certainly top of mind while pushing. The fear of tearing is totally understandable, and it's a topic that comes up a lot in prenatal conversations. Moms, whether they choose medication or not, also tend to stress about feeling the tear happening. The good news is that with all the other sensations you're feeling during labor, noticing the tear itself is not very common. Besides that, there's the whole postpartum recovery to think about, which can be a bit nerve-wracking, especially when it involves healing after a tear. But, rest assured, there are ways to ease these worries and make the whole experience a bit smoother.

The degree of a tear ranges from first-degree, which involves minor tearing of the vaginal lining, to fourth-degree, which extends into the muscles and through the anal sphincter. Most common is the second-degree tear, especially for a first time mom, which is a little deeper than a surface tear, with some muscle being affected. Most providers will recommend a repair for anything beyond a skin or surface tear.

Tips that can help prevent tears

To help prevent tearing during pushing, consider the following tips:

Perineal Massage: Gently massaging the perineal area during the last few weeks of pregnancy to increase its flexibility and reduce the risk of tearing.

Squats: Doing squats prenatally can help strengthen the pelvic floor muscles in a way that helps reduce tears. Adding squatting each time you bend down to pick something up in the 3rd trimester can help you incorporate squats in your everyday life.

Warm Compresses: Applying warm compresses to the perineum during the pushing stage to soften the tissue and make it more pliable. Ask the care team if they have warmers they can use as warm compresses, if not, a bin of wash clothes in hot water work well too.

Slow and Controlled Pushing: Pushing slowly and controlled during contractions, rather than forcefully, can decrease the risk of tearing. Some mom's find using a mirror to see (especially with an epidural) can help them be more effective and more controlled with pushing.

Positioning: Experiment with different pushing positions, such as side-lying, which may reduce pressure on the perineum.

Use a Mirror: Slowing down right as baby is crowning helps minimize tearing. Being able to see, using a mirror, can really help with knowing when and how to slow down.

Hydration and Nutrition: Staying well-hydrated and maintaining proper nutrition prenatally can help keep the tissues in the perineal area healthy and resilient.

Breathing Techniques: Utilize proper breathing techniques during pushing to avoid overbearing down on the perineum.

Episiotomy Consideration: Discuss the necessity of an episiotomy (a surgical cut) with your healthcare provider, as it may help reduce severe tears in some cases.

Effective Communication: Communicate openly with your healthcare team and birth support about your comfort, sensations, and preferences during pushing.

Prenatal Care: Discussions with your healthcare provider about your birthing plan can help address any concerns about tearing and help you come up with a plan to support your perineum during pushing.

Follow Postpartum Care: Adhering to recommended postpartum care, such as gentle cleansing and perineal care, can promote healing after childbirth.

Pelvic Floor Therapy: Seeking out pelvic floor therapy after your postpartum period can play a huge role in long term recovery and pelvic floor strength and health.

When does tearing happen?

Many mom's worry about tearing so much that they are reluctant and hold back while pushing. It's important to understand that tearing only happens as baby is crowning and with baby's body being born. Until baby's head is crowning you are safe to push with all the strength, power, and force you have and not worry about tearing. Your provider team will help you know when it's time to slow down to avoid tearing; until than, there is no need to hold back.

Using gravity — standing, squatting or hands-and-knees — is so helpful in the pushing stage to encourage baby's descent and movement passed the pubic bone. However, gravity can increase the chance of tearing as it adds extra pressure on your pelvic floor muscles and adds more force to your pushing. A suggestion you may consider is using gravity for the first part of your pushing stage, and then moving to a side-lying or back position to push as baby is crowning and being born.

Anecdotally, when a provider manually assists or guides a baby out once the head is born, pulling the baby out instead of letting the baby be born naturally, the chance of tearing can increase. To prevent tears from a providers manual guidance at delivery, you can request to wait for the next contraction once baby's head is born, and with the next contraction you gently, and with control birth the rest of your baby's body. If this is something you would prefer, have a conversation with your provider before birth, have it written in your birth plan, and communicate it before you start pushing. If there is a medical necessity for added guidance and support from your provider as the baby is being born, of course, you would trust and lean on your provider to make that decision in the moment. Choosing a provider you feel confident with and trust, who's philosophy aligns with yours makes a huge difference in this decision and many others in your birth.

It's not very common to feel the pain of the tear as it is happening. With all the other pressure and stretching sensations the tear often is unnoticed in the moment it is occurring. It's when your provider does a vaginal check after birth that you get a clear assessment if you have torn and to what degree.

Even with all the intentional prenatal prep, perineal massages, and controlled pushing sometimes a tear may be inevitable. The way baby stretches and moves through your birth canal and comes through at birth can cause an internal vaginal tear that cannot be prevented with these techniques. Internal vaginal tears are repaired by your provider immediately postpartum and often don't cause the same stinging and discomfort an external tear can.

Perineal Stretching & Massage

Perineal stretching and massage during the pushing stage of labor are techniques intended to reduce or minimize the risk of tearing. When done correctly, they can increase the flexibility of the perineal tissues, making them more pliable and less likely to tear as the baby's head passes through the birth canal. These techniques aim to gently prepare and ease the perineum for the stretching it will naturally undergo during childbirth.

The key here is, if they are done correctly. While research on the effectiveness of perineal stretching and massage during the pushing stage is mixed, many healthcare providers recommend these practices as they can potentially reduce the likelihood of severe tears. According to studies, perineal massaging and stretching can be effective in reducing tears if the provider does them properly and has a reliable track record of reduced tearing with their aid. This can be a great conversation to have with your provider prenatally.

Studies have proven that perineal massage prenatally, in the weeks before labor, can be effective in reducing tears.

Ultimately, the impact of perineal stretching and massage prenatally and while pushing can vary from person to person, and it may not entirely eliminate the risk of tearing, but it's considered a helpful strategy to potentially reduce the severity of tears during childbirth. If you prefer to not have perineal massage during pushing, you would have to communicate that clearly with your provider team before and during pushing.

Utilizing these prevention tips can help avoid a tear or at least have a tear that is only a one or two degree tear rather than a more severe tear. Healthcare providers are experienced in managing and repairing tears when necessary and will do repairs immediately after delivery. Open communication with your healthcare team is vital, as they can provide guidance on the best strategies to prevent and address tearing during childbirth.

10

What If I Need A C-section?

Avoiding a C-section is often on the top of most mom's priority list of wishes and preferences for birth. Mom's often try to plan all of their birth decisions around ensuring they can achieve a vaginal birth. So, are there any methods or approaches that can help avoid a C-section?

L abor can be filled with unplanned and unexpected twists and turns, and sometimes, a cesarean section, often referred to as a C-section, becomes an unexpected but medically necessary part of the path. In this chapter, we'll explore the step-by-step process of a C-section, the range of emotions that you may experience, and the pivotal role that a support team plays in providing comfort and guidance throughout this unique birthing experience. If a C-section becomes necessary for you, the hope is that this information will help you feel less overwhelm and fear. Having a basic understanding and knowledge of what is happening with your body and your baby during a C-section can help you feel more at ease in the process.

The Step-by-Step Process

A cesarean section is a surgical procedure in which a baby is delivered through an incision made in the abdomen and uterus. While every C-section experience may vary slightly, the following steps provide a general overview of what to anticipate:

Preparation: Prior to the surgery, you will be prepped and brought into the operating room. The prep includes giving you a bag of fluids through your IV, administered antibiotics and anti-nausea medications, and oral pain medications. If needed, a nurse will shave the area where the incision will be made.

Pain Management: Once in the operating room; an epidural or spinal block is administered to ensure you are pain-free during the procedure while allowing you to remain awake and alert. Most often, you are brought into the OR alone, prepped, and then your partner and doula join you just before the surgery begins.

Drape: A drape is placed just above your chest so you and your partner do not see any of the surgery. Some hospitals offer a clear drape to see your baby immediately after born. A dark drape is placed on during the surgery and then dropped to the clear drape once your baby is born.

Incision: The area where the incision is made is sterilized with a sterile solution and a clear drape is placed on your belly to maintain the sterile field. The surgeon will make a horizontal incision just above your pubic bone. In some cases, a vertical incision may be necessary.

Uterine Incision: Following the abdominal incision, a uterine incision is made to access the baby. The type of uterine incision (usually a low transverse incision) may vary based on factors such as the baby's position.

Delivery: The baby is carefully delivered from the uterus. The pediatric team will be on standby to attend to your newborn's needs.

Baby Care: Once baby is born, typically a 60 sec delayed cord clamping occurs, then the provider cuts cord and hands baby off to the baby care team. Some providers will place your baby onto your chest immediately through the drape before the cord is clamped. Baby is taken to a warmer and assessed and any needed medical support is provided.

Placental Removal: After the baby is safely delivered, the placenta is removed, and the surgeon will perform all necessary repairs, such as closing the uterine incision.

Closure: The surgeon closes the abdominal incision layer by layer, typically with dissolvable sutures. Staples or external sutures may also be used.

Recovery: You will be transferred to a recovery room where you will be closely monitored as you wake from the anesthesia. Once stable, you'll be reunited with your baby in most cases. Some baby's remain with mom in the OR and mom and baby are transported to recovery together.

Family-centered C-sections

In many hospitals you can request a family-centered C-section which will prioritize (if medically possible) that you and your baby remain together, have a clear drape to see baby immediately, delayed cord clamping for baby, skin-to-skin in the OR, and an opportunity to nurse as soon as possible. You can specify all these preferences to your provider team before your C-section (assuming it is not emergent).

Most C-sections are not an emergency, which gives you time to ask questions of your provider, be walked through the surgical procedure, and have some time to process and space to feel the emotions that come with this big shift. You can always request a few minutes to just be with your partner and let the news sink in before you move forward with a non-emergent C-section.

Emotional Aspects of C-sections

A C-section can be an emotionally complex experience. It's not uncommon for you to feel a range of emotions, including disappointment, fear, sadness, or even relief. This reaction is entirely normal, as C-sections often deviate from the envisioned birth plan. It's helpful to remember that when a C-section occurs, it is a valid and necessary method of birthing, serving the best interests of both you and your baby.

As a doula, I've witnessed firsthand the importance of emotional support during a C-section. My role goes beyond physical comfort; it includes providing reassurance, helping you understand the process, and encouraging open communication with the medical team. Your doula will be there to remind you that your journey into parenthood, while different from what you expected, is just as valid and beautiful.

Your Support Team's Vital Role

Your birthing experience is a profound moment of your life and a C-section doesn't shortchange that in any way. Your support team plays a pivotal role in ensuring you feel comforted and informed. Here's how your partner, doula and other support members can help:

Emotional Support: Your doula provides a listening ear, offering a safe space for you to express your feelings and concerns. A doula acknowledges the significance of your emotions and helps you navigate them with understanding and empathy.

Education: A doula can help demystify the surgical process by explaining each step in a clear, reassuring manner. Knowing what to expect can alleviate anxiety and provide a sense of control.

Advocacy: Your doula advocates for your birthing preferences, working in harmony with the medical team to ensure your choices are respected whenever possible. They help you sustain your voice when you may feel vulnerable.

Comfort Techniques: Even in the operating room, comfort techniques such as deep breathing, guided visualization, and gentle touch can be employed to help you stay relaxed and grounded. Playing music and using essential oils can help set the environment to give you a sense of comfort and excitement to meet your baby in the moment.

Immediate Bonding: Your support team can facilitate the earliest moments of bonding by ensuring your baby is placed on your chest as soon as possible, encouraging skin-to-skin contact and helping with breastfeeding.

Postpartum Care: Following the birth, your doula can assist with post-operative care, supporting you as you begin your recovery journey and adjusting to your new role as a parent in light of having surgery.

Remember, a C-section doesn't in any way diminish the strength, courage, or love that you bring to this transformative moment in your life. Your birth story is uniquely yours, and with the unwavering support of your entire birth team, it can be a beautifully empowering and memorable start into parenthood.

11

Welcoming Your Birth

Getting a deeper understanding of the stages of labor and the coping techniques that help you navigate each of the stages, from early contractions to the triumphant moment of birth, will serve as an invaluable guide that will keep you feeling confidence and courageous throughout your labor. Together, we've explored the intricate dance of body, mind, and heart, uncovering the tools, techniques, and rhythms that can empower you during this incredible journey of childbirth.

As your virtual birth doula, I've walked alongside you, sharing insights and strategies to help you embrace this life-changing experience. Now, as we wrap, it's essential to recognize that every labor is unique, just as every birth story is unique. Your body, mind, and heart will act as your most reliable companions, ensuring a profound connection to your labor experience.

I want you to carry this message with you: You are strong. You are capable. You are the author of your birth story. With the rhythms and affirmations you've cultivated, you hold the key to navigate your birth experience with confidence, resilience, and grace.

This isn't just about coping with labor; it's about thriving in the process. The tools and insights we've shared are your birthright, your sources of empowerment. Whether your labor is swift or meandering, intense or gentle, medicated or unmedicated, know that your journey is your own, and you are fully equipped to embrace it.

As you move forward on this incredible path towards childbirth, remember that your birth team, whether in-person or in spirit, is here to support you, lift you, and empower you. Each contraction, each surge, brings you closer to meeting your little one, and it's a moment you're beautifully poised to embrace.

Trust in your body, trust in your heart, trust in your mind. You've got this, and your birth story is waiting to be written – with strength, resilience, and, most of all, love.

Here's to the remarkable and beautiful journey ahead – your birth, your story, your power.

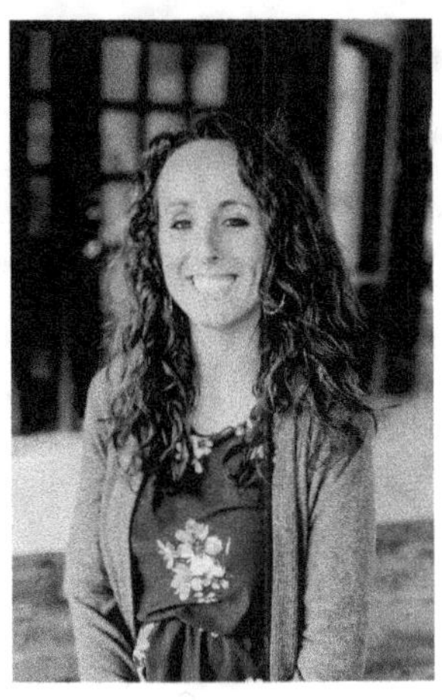

About the Author

Ema, a dedicated birth and postpartum doula, brings her invaluable personal experience as a mother of three to her role as the founder and owner of Empowered Birthing Doula Services in vibrant Nashville, Tennessee. With a deep-seated belief that every mom-to-be possesses an innate capacity and strength to navigate birth with confidence and courage, Ema is on a mission to transform the birthing narrative from fear to freedom. Her passion for providing the right resources and unwavering support shines through in her work, and this guide is a testament to her commitment to empower every expectant mother and their partner, equipping them to embrace the beauty of their birth experience with confidence and joy.

You can connect with me on:

🌐 https://www.ebdoula.com

f https://www.instagram.com/empowered_birthing